Copyright

Get Spartan Shredded: How to Build a Muscular Ripped Physique like a 300 Warrior

March 2014

Scott James

www.Shredded-Society.com

Disclaimer

The information provided in this book is designed to provide helpful information on the subjects discussed. This book is not meant to be used, nor should it be used, to diagnose or treat any medical condition. For diagnosis or treatment of any medical problem, consult your own physician. The publisher and author are not responsible for any specific health or allergy needs that may require medical supervision and are not liable for any damages or negative consequences from any treatment, action, application or preparation, to any person reading or following the information in this book. References are provided for informational purposes only and do not constitute endorsement of any websites or other sources. Readers should be aware that the websites listed in this book may change.

I recommend consulting a doctor to assess and/or identify any health related issues prior to making any dramatic changes to your diet and/or exercise regime.

Contents

About the Author

Scott James has been addicted to all things fitness, health and nutrition for nearly a decade.

With a large amount of hype surrounding the fitness industry, as well as the dieting and supplementation niches Scott thought it was the right time to come forward and debunk the myths and scams within the industry.

All information conveyed in Scott's books is tried and tested - no false hope or bad information is shared.

Scott believes that when an individual is equipped with the correct knowledge and a plan of action that he will provide in his books they are unstoppable.

Scott is not here to make money, he's here to make a different and guide you on your journey to unlocking the new, better you.

Intro

I want to thank you and congratulate you for downloading 'Get Spartan Shredded.'

In this book, you will learn exactly how to achieve a shredded Spartan-like physique with immense strength.

Your new found body will command attention and respect; you'll have an aura around you. Girls will want you and guys will want to know your secret.

Throw your old exercise regime and diet out the window and prepare to be introduced to a training philosophy that is not only straight to the point and easy to follow but also delivers immense results.

This book comprehensively covers everything from the routines to follow, with a breakdown of each and every individual exercise, a complete shredded Spartan abdominal annihilation regime, a comprehensive diet planning chapter, including how to know exactly how much to eat in order to get utterly shredded or stack on tons of quality lean muscle mass, a look into how to stay motivated and how to continually track your progress to ensure you are on the path to success.

Should you choose to follow the principles I have documented for you in this book, you'll not only build the body of your dreams, but you will also unknowingly build unbreakable confidence, pride and determination. Your mind will reflect your body and you will be unstoppable – any dreams, goals, or aspirations you have will suddenly all be within reach.

Thanks again for downloading this book, I hope you enjoy it!

Bonus Content

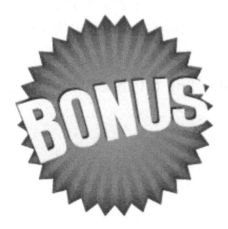

As a token of my appreciation I would like to give you access to my exclusive bonus content.

<u>You're only a click away from receiving:</u>

Exclusive pre-release access to my latest eBooks

Free eBooks during promotional periods

Simply navigate to http://shredded-society.com/Spartan.html

In order to receive this bonus content.

As this is a limited time offer it would be a shame to miss out, I recommend grabbing these bonuses at your earliest convenience.

Why You Should Become a Spartan Warrior

Go to your local shopping mall, go to the movies, go anywhere out in public and tell me what you see.

You see skinny, frail, effeminate looking men with low testosterone. Are you one of them? If you are, I can guarantee you won't be for much longer...

As we don't live in the Spartan era – we don't have to hunt for our food all day with spears and crossbows. Everything is provided to us, and we have become far too comfortable and reliant upon society for nutrition.

However, YOU are about to separate yourself from that pack of sheep - **you're about to become a lion amongst the sheep, you are about to become a Spartan Warrior.**

In order to become a real man, raise your testosterone and separate yourself from the 'nobodies' in this world, you join the gym, pack on masses of lean muscle, become immensely stronger, and you torch all that fat you have accrued.

You've now acquired the mindset of a true Spartan Warrior (aka a winner in this world).

'Don't judge a book by its cover' – a saying as old as the hills. I'm sure your parents have told you this, and I'm sure this saying was drilled into your head in elementary school. I'm here to tell you that Spartans DO judge others by their physical appearance. Spartans look down upon those members of society who have been given just one body and choose to neglect it by never exercising or eating correctly. Everybody has the opportunity to be great, yet sadly so few choose to take it.

Let's take a look at a few examples of 'judging a book by its cover':

Stand next to the most muscular guy you can find. Now how do you feel?

Are you intimidated? *Yes...*

Do you feel that he is better and stronger than you? *Yes...*

Do you feel he has pride and confidence in himself? *Yes...*

Do you think he is successful in his other endeavours outside of the gym? *Yes...*

Does he have a winner's mentality? *Yes...*

Now, after you've done that, stand next to the skinniest guy you can find:
Now how do you feel?

Do you feel that he is better and stronger than you? *Nope...*

Do you feel he has pride and confidence in himself? *Nope...*

Do you think he is successful in his other endeavours outside of the gym? *Nope...*

Does he have a winner's mentality? *Nope...*

BOOM! You just judged those two individuals by their physical appearance, aka their 'cover.' See? Everybody does it, and it does seem to be quite accurate.

The below photo displays my own 30 month transformation. By looking at the photo, you can clearly tell I added in excess of 20kg of lean muscle mass. What you can't see is the mental transformation that also took place, which is far more powerful than the addition of any muscle.

I gained confidence.

I learned to love the process.

I began to take pride in all of my endeavours, not just in the gym.

I stopped being a talker, I became a walker.

I became a Shredded Spartan, both physically and mentally.

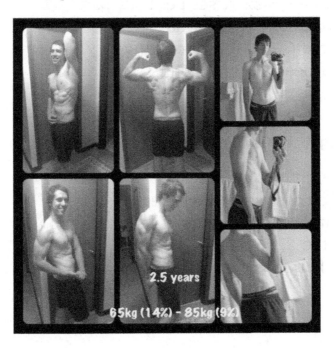

Strength vs. Size

If you've ever read a fitness magazine or spent time browsing the internet trying to find out how to pack on muscle, get ripped and gain strength, I'm sure you would've encountered the two opposing parties: those that recommend to train like a bodybuilder in order to get big, and those that tell you to train less frequently for pure strength, which supposedly results in huge muscle mass gains.

Let's take a look at both:

Bodybuilding:

Train 5/6 times per week
Perform 4 – 6 exercises per body part
Train one body part per day
Lift in the 6 – 12 repetition range
Lift reasonably light weights

Strength Training:

Train 3/4 times per week
Focus on compound exercises
Perform full body exercises each session
Lift in the 1 – 6 repetition range
Lift as heavy as possible

I DO NOT RECOMMEND YOU FOLLOW EITHER OF THESE CONVENTIONAL ROUTES.

Here's why...

Bodybuilding magazines (I'm not going to name names here) give you two-thirds of the equation; they share a workout routine and a diet consisting of ~6 meals of chicken and rice along with a few protein shakes throughout the day, which is all well and good, but they fail to mention that in order to pack on size and strength following one of these low weight, high repetition style workout regimes, you need to be injecting a cocktail of anabolic compounds (which are not exactly healthy).

Conventional strength training (programs such as Rippetoes, Stronglifts and Westside for Skinny Bastards) rely on the human body to operate like a piece of machinery in order to progress – the weight you are going to lift is calculated far in advance, which is based off a certain percentage of your 1RM (1 rep maximum for that particular exercise). Unfortunately, the human body doesn't exact operate like a machine. Some days you will be feeling more energised, and as a result you will be able to lift the prescribed weight. Other times you may fail – that's just how the human body is... strength gain is not necessarily always linear.

Yes, you will gain strength through a strength training program, but you will not gain the bulging chest, thick vascular arms or tight, shredded abs that you desire simply due to the low amount of volume included in these routines. People who train specifically for strength are forever afraid of 'over training.' In order to build a Spartan-like physique, a certain amount of volume is required, which is something a solely strength based routine cannot provide you.

Here's how you become Spartan Shredded

In order to become Spartan Shredded while staying natural (not relying on any anabolic compounds, aka steroids), a certain balance between strength training and bodybuilding must be accomplished. You're going to be training with a base of strength exercises – the essentials such as the squat, bench, deadlift and overhead press in which you will be lifting heavy for few repetitions. Assistance exercises are implemented in higher volume, a range of around 6 – 12 repetitions, in order to take your muscles to the hypertrophy stage, allowing you to pack on size by exhausting and destroying the muscle.

Training Volume

As a beginner, I recommend working out four days per week. Once your body begins to adapt to this volume of training, you can increase your training regime to 5-6 sessions per week provided your body is able to recover effectively in time (this comes down to correct nutrition, rest and supplementation).

Ask anyone with a notable physique how often they workout – I can guarantee the answer will be either 5 or 6 days per week. If you want to get serious results, you must have a serious training regime.

Working out must become a habit, just like brushing your teeth in the morning and eating your meals. If you really want it, you'll make time in your day. If not, you'll make an excuse.

Results or excuses – choose one... you can't have both.

Perhaps you've read a fitness magazine or spoken to other gym-goers who have warned you about the dreaded 'overtraining' that can occur if you train more than four days per week. I guarantee you those who whine and moan about 'overtraining' are either:

Not seeing results because they aren't following a well-designed workout regime

Or

Too lazy to spend additional time at the gym; they'd rather be at home relaxing (claiming that they would overtrain if they went more frequently as the perfect excuse).

If you're smart about your training and follow the structured Spartan routine I present to you later in this book, get enough sleep each night and consume an adequate amount of calories daily, the thought of overtraining will never even cross your mind.

Each of your training sessions should last between 45 minutes and an hour, any less time and you won't be able to get in the necessary volume to make the workout worthwhile, and any longer than an hour means your training intensity is far too low – your rest between sets should be 1 minute for your main strength exercises and 30 – 45 seconds for your assistance (isolation) exercises.

You're not at the gym to make new friends and chit chat about the weather. You get in, do your workout, and get out - Spartans are efficient.

The Shredded Spartan Workout Regime

The Shredded Spartan Workout Regime is based around four main exercises. These include:

Bench Press

Squat

Deadlift

Overhead Press

IT ALL STARTS HERE
If you want to get big and strong, you're going to have to master these first.

The above eight exercises form the basis of any workout regime.
All other exercises are essentially a variation of these exercises. For example: an incline dumbbell press is a variation of the bench press, dumbbell Arnold presses are a variation of the traditional overhead press, meanwhile one legged split squats are a variation of the barbell squat.

The Shredded Spartan Workout Regime will have you performing each of the above exercises a minimum of once per week and a maximum of three times per week.

Each muscle group (e.g. chest, back, shoulders, arms, legs) will be trained a minimum of once per week and a maximum of three times per week.

The more stimulation each muscle group gets the better. The usual one body part once per week style bodybuilding routine just isn't going to cut it if you want a god-like Spartan physique.

Workout Structure

The Shredded Spartan workout regime isn't rocket science. You won't have to remember a vast number of complex exercises or calculate weight percentages between your sets. The Spartans were strong and efficient in all their endeavours... this routine reflects that.

Each of your workouts will consist of:

1 or 2 main exercises (heavy, low repetition)

2 – 4 assistance exercises (lighter, high repetition)

As mentioned previously, by combining these heavy main lifts with higher repetition isolation exercises, this will allow you to acquire both the strength and size you're after.

Super-human strength or shredded abs?

Why choose when you can have both?!

The Main Lifts

The following exercises are categorised as our main lifts. These exercises are going to be performed heavy for a few repetitions in order to build your foundation of strength.

Chest

Barbell Bench Press

Back

Conventional Deadlifts

Shoulders

Barbell Overhead Press

Legs

Barbell Back Squats

Your main lifts are to be performed at the beginning of your workout, before any assistance work. You will be performing 5 sets consisting of 3 – 5 repetitions for your main lifts – you will be pyramiding up in weight and down in repetitions. Let's take a look at an example of your bench press main lift:

Set 1 – 150lbs – 5 reps

Set 2 - 165lbs – 5 reps

Set 3 – 180lbs – 4 reps

Set 4 – 190lbs - 4 reps

Set 5 – 205lbs – 3 reps

As we're primarily working on building our strength with these main lifts, the primary focus is on going as heavy as you possibly can while still obtaining between 3 and 5 repetitions with strict form.

Assistance Work

The following exercises are designed to achieve muscular hypertrophy – these are to be performed after your initial 1 – 2 heavy, low repetition main compound exercises.

The primary purpose of these exercises is to add shape and size to your muscles, so these exercises should be performed slowly with reasonably light weight. You are to focus on the extension and contraction of the muscle; think about the muscle as it moves to really engage the 'mind-muscle' connection.

Chest

Incline Dumbbell Press
Incline Dumbbell flyes
Cable Crossovers

Back

Pull-ups
Lat Pulldowns
Bent Over Rows

Shoulders

Arnold Presses
Dumbbell Lateral Raises
Dumbbell Rear Deltoid Flies

Arms

Barbell Curls
Incline Dumbbell Curls

Barbell Skullcrushers
Tricep Dips

Legs

Leg Press
Leg Extensions
Straight Leg Deadlift

Your assistance exercises are to be performed after you have completed all of your main lifts for that particular session - not before.

As mentioned above, you are to disregard heavy weight on your assistance exercise – these are to shape and fatigue the muscle. In order to do that, we need to work within a higher repetition range (8-12), practise strict form (no jerking, swinging, half repetitions or using momentum to get the weight up), and go slow on the negative (eccentric) portion of each repetition.

Assistance exercises are to be performed on an as-needed basis. This is referred to as 'Priority Training' as each individual has different strong, lagging and genetically superior muscle groups. Perhaps you were blessed with broad shoulders, but your arms are quite skinny... in this case, you will place on an emphasis on your arm training by selecting exercises out of the 'Arms' assistance exercise category several times per week.

Exercise Explanations

On the following page, you will find an explanation of each exercise. These exercises are categorised into:

Main Lifts

Assistance Exercises – Chest

Assistance Exercises – Back

Assistance Exercises – Shoulders

Assistance Exercises – Arms

Assistance Exercises – Legs

Main Lifts

The Squat

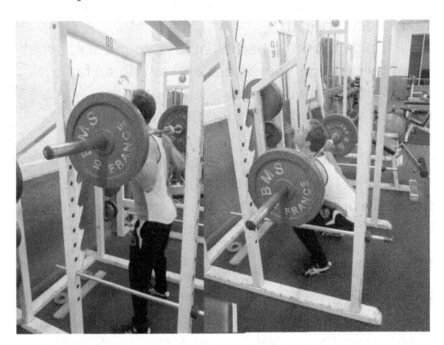

Muscles Worked:

Quads, calves, glute, hamstrings, lower back

Description:

The barbell squat will singlehandedly transform your body. Squats are included in every exercise regime whether you're looking to gain mass, increase your leg power for sports or even for injury rehabilitation and prevention. Without a doubt, the squat is the king of all exercises.

Form:

Use a slightly wider than shoulder-width stance.
Take a deep breath.
While holding onto a barbell across your back, squat down by bending your knees and sitting as far back as possible with your hips.
Look forward to ensure your lower back does not round.
Once you have reached an angle at which your legs are parallel to the floor, push through your heels and exhale in order to return to the starting position.
Repeat for the prescribed number of repetitions (5).

Common Mistakes:

Ensure you are reaching parallel; you are only cheating yourself by performing partial repetitions (partial repetitions will only work the quads, while deep squats will engage your hamstrings and glutes).

Look straight ahead; do not look down as you will begin to round your lower back, leaving you extremely vulnerable to injury.

Ensure you are driving backwards with your hips; many beginners attempt to lean forward when squatting, and in doing so they are unable to get the required depth and they are pushing through their toes, quite often with their heel off the ground – this all comes down to practise.

The Bench

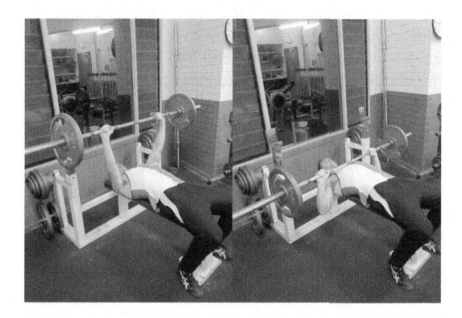

Muscles Worked:

Chest, shoulders, triceps

Description:

The bench press, the exercise males most commonly refer to as a measure of strength, is a fantastic upper body compound exercise that will primarily blast the chest, but will also assist with adding mass to your shoulders and triceps as they are the secondary muscle groups recruited while performing the flat barbell bench press.

Form:

Lie comfortably on a flat bench.
Utilise a medium grip, slightly outside of shoulder width.
Exhale and unrack the bar and begin to lower it to the middle of your chest, stopping just before the barbell touches your chest.
Exhale and drive the barbell upwards while focusing on your chest muscles, then contract your chest by squeezing at the top of each repetition.
Repeat for the prescribed number of repetitions (5).

Common Mistakes:

Ensure you are lowering the bar to an inch above your chest level - do not cheat by performing partial repetitions.

On the other extreme, do not bounce the barbell off your chest. Many people do this when lifting heavy – by relying on the momentum to complete each repetition you may be able to move the weight, but you certainly won't be gaining the full benefit as the 'bounce' is taking tension off your muscles.

Ensure your feet are touching the floor, bring them in as close to the bench as possible. (Ever notice how Olympic lifters keep their legs as close to the bench as possible, creating a slight arch in their back? This is correct form and it will help you lift more!) Many beginners neglect this fact and instead take their feet off the floor as they begin to struggle, which makes the bench press slightly harder than it already is.

The Deadlift

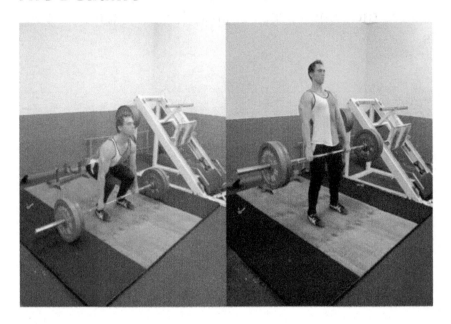

Muscles Worked:

Lower back, calves, forearms, glutes, hamstrings, lats, middle back, quads, traps

Description:

The barbell deadlift is the king of all exercises. If you told me you only had time to perform one exercise, I would tell you to deadlift! The deadlift is a complete body workout; essentially all muscles in the body are recruited when performing a conventional deadlift. Many individuals get scared at the thought of the deadlift, but provided your form is correct and you start off light, you will not encounter any issues.

Form:

Stand in front of your barbell with a shoulder width stance.

Bend your knees while keeping your back straight in order to get down and grip the barbell with your choice of either a double overhand or a mixed (one overhand, one underhand) grip.

Push through your heels while straightening your upper body in order to get the barbell off the ground.

Exhale as you protrude your chest forward while pulling your shoulder blades back to complete the repetition.

Bend your knees and lean forward while keeping a straight back to return the barbell to the ground.

Repeat for the prescribed number of repetitions (5).

Common Mistakes:

There is no way physically possible to cheat on a deadlift, the weight is dead on the ground – you have to pick it up from a stationary position.

Ensure your back is straight as you pull the deadlift. If your back is beginning to round while you are struggling to lock out the weight, this indicates it is too heavy and you're at a high risk of injuring your lower back. In this case, my only recommendation is to lower the weight until you are strong enough to attempt that weight again.

When performing subsequent repetitions, ensure you are not bouncing the barbell off the ground. Lower the bar to the ground until it is completely stationary before performing your next repetition.

The Barbell Overhead Press

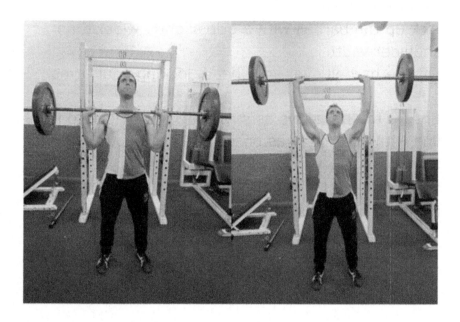

Muscles Worked:

Shoulders, chest, triceps

Description:

The barbell overhead press is a monster mass builder for your shoulders. If you want cannonball shaped deltoids, this is the way to get them! The barbell shoulder press can be performed standing or seated, both will work the shoulders in the same fashion (although standing will also utilise your core to stabilise the weight).

Form:

Start with the barbell loaded on a rack just around neck/head height.
Pick up the barbell with a grip slightly wider than shoulder width.
Lift the barbell over your head, locking your arms out.
Ensure the bar stays as straight and as close to in line with your body as possible – push up, don't push forwards.
Lower the bar slowly back down to the starting position.

Common Mistakes:

Many beginners grip the bar far too narrow; this places too much emphasis on the triceps as opposed to the shoulders.

For the most efficient movement, keep the bar as close to your body as possible. Many beginners push the barbell forwards unknowingly while they are lifting it up.

Do not cheat the repetitions. If you are doing standing barbell overhead press by pushing through your legs, this is referred to as a push press. Yes, this exercise has a time and place, but you're here to build pure shoulder strength via strict form overhead press, not to perform a push press.

Assistance Exercises – Chest

Incline Dumbbell Press

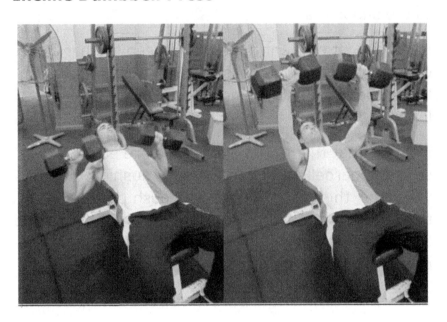

Description:

The incline dumbbell press targets the upper thickness of the chest.

Form:

Lie on an incline bench set at a 30 degree angle. Load the dumbbells up to the starting position by pushing them off your thighs.
Once the dumbbells are up at shoulder width, ensure your palms are facing away from you.
Lower the dumbbells until they touch your chest.

Exhale as you begin to push the dumbbells back up –
completing the repetition when your arms lock out.
Hold at the top of the movement for 1 second,
squeezing your chest to contract.
Repeat for desired number of repetitions (8-12).

Incline Dumbbell Flyes

Description:

Incline dumbbell flyes assist in building the width of
your upper chest.

Form:

Lie on an incline bench set at a 30 degree angle.
Load the dumbbells up to the starting position by
pushing them off your thighs.
Once the dumbbells are up at shoulder width, ensure
your palms are facing each other.
Proceed to lower the dumbbells to your side while
keeping a slight bend in your arm.
Lower the dumbbell as far as possible and hold for a
moment to stretch the chest.
Return the dumbbell to their starting position by
pushing up while still maintaining that bend in your
arms.
Repeat for the desired number of repetitions (8-12).

NOTE: The best way to get the motion (while
maintaining bent arms) correct is to imagine you are
hugging a large tree. As strange as that sounds, I
have been able to teach individuals good form

consistently by preaching this analogy.

Cable Crossovers

Description:

Cable crossovers assist in developing primarily the width of the chest, but will also aid with chest thickness too. The higher the cable pulleys are set, the more upper chest is worked. If the pulleys are set around shoulder width height, you will hit more of the middle chest. Likewise, setting the cable pulleys low will emphasize the lower chest.

Form:

Take several large steps forward from the cable machine with one handle of the cables in each hand. Slightly bend your torso forward.
With a slight bend in your arms, just like with dumbbells, bring the handles of the cables together, contracting your chest in the middle while holding onto the handles in front of you.
Proceed to extend your arms to the side in an arc until you feel a deep stretch in your chest.
Return to the starting position while maintaining a bend in your arms.
Repeat for the desired number of repetitions (8-12).

Assistance Exercises – Back

Pull-ups

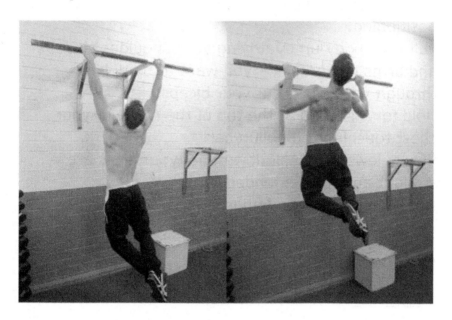

Description:

The pullup is an exceptional exercise for adding mass and width to the upper back and biceps, and it is great for measuring strength in comparison to bodyweight. Ignite new growth into your lats with wide grip pull-ups. Once you've mastered sets of 12 bodyweight pull-ups, it's time to start adding additional resistance.

Form:

Using a wider than shoulder width grip, grasp the pullup bar with palms facing away from you.
Push your chest forward and curve your lower back slightly backwards to create a slight angle in your positioning.
Pull your body up by driving your shoulder blades and arms down/back – you want to be pulling through your back, not your biceps.
Hold for 1 second at the top of the rep with your chest touching the pullup bar.
Slowly lower yourself down until your arms are straight and fully extended.
Repeat for desired number of repetitions (8-12).

Lat Pulldowns

Description:

The lat pulldown, just like the pullup, is fantastic for developing overall back width.
By increasing your lat pulldown, your ability to perform pull-ups will increase greatly.

Form:

Sit down on a lat pulldown machine, lock your knees in, and grasp the bar with a wider than shoulder width grip with palms facing away from you.
Push your chest forward and curve your lower back slightly backwards to create a slight angle in your positioning.
Pull the bar down by driving your shoulder blades

and arms back/down – you want be pulling through your lats as opposed to your biceps.

Hold for 1 second to contract your back muscles. Return the bar to its starting positioning by straightening your arms.

Maintain the slightly angled position for the entire duration of your set - don't rock backwards and forwards between repetitions.

Repeat for desired number of repetitions (8-12).

Bent Over Rows

Description:

The bent over barbell row will add thickness to your middle back; we can place greater emphasis on the inner, middle, and outer back thickness by adjusting our grip placement on the barbell. Bent over rows also heavily utilise the abdominal muscles and lower back in order to stabilise the weight.

Form:

Grasp a barbell with your palms facing down.
Bend your knees and bring your body forwards, bend at the waist and maintain a straight back while attempting to maintain a position as parallel to the floor as possible.
While keeping your body in this position, pull the barbell towards you by pulling your shoulder blades together.
Pull the barbell upwards and back towards your belly button.
Hold and squeeze in position for 1 second, focusing on the middle back.
Breathe in and lower the barbell back to the ground (do not touch the ground).
Repeat for desired number of repetitions (8-12).

Assistance Exercises – Shoulders

Arnold Press

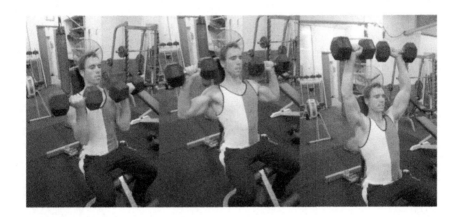

Description:

The Arnold Press has been used to add that rounded shape and make the shoulders 'pop' for years, first made famous by Arnold Schwarzenegger, the legend himself. The rotation during the Arnold Press ensures that all heads of the shoulder are hit during each repetition.

Form:

Sit on a bench with adequate back support, with your dumbbells seated on your knees.
Raise the dumbbells to chest level with palms facing towards you.
Raise the dumbbell and rotate your palms until they are facing forward.

Pause at the top for 1 second.
Lower the dumbbells to chest level, rotating your palms until they are facing towards you again.
Perform for the desired number of repetitions (8-12).

Dumbbell Lateral Raises

Description:

Dumbbell side lateral raises are a fantastic isolation exercise for the shoulders; the side lateral raise specifically targets the medial (side) portion of the shoulder. Focus on slow, controlled form while performing side lateral raises, and watch your medial deltoids begin to explode with width and thickness.

Form:

Stand straight with a very slight behind in your knees.
Keep the dumbbells by your sides with palms also facing your sides.
With a slight bend in the arm and with your hands slightly tilted forwards, begin to lift the dumbbells until your arms are parallel to the floor. At the top of each repetition, tilt your hands down slightly as if you were pouring a jug of water.
Lower the dumbbells slowly back down to your sides.
Repeat for desired number of repetitions (8-12).

Dumbbell Rear Deltoid Flies

Description:

Dumbbell rear deltoid flies focus on adding mass and definition to the rear deltoid (the rear portion of your shoulders). The rear deltoid is often neglected, as it is rarely seen. It is crucial to hit all heads of the deltoid evenly to maintain proportion and symmetry; the key to the ultimate Spartan body is the right balance between size, symmetry and proportions of the muscle.

Form:

Lay face down on a flat bench, holding a dumbbell in each hand with palms facing towards each other. With your elbows maintaining a slight bend, raise your arms until your elbows are at your shoulder height. At this point your arms should be roughly parallel to the ground.
Hold this position for one moment, squeezing your shoulder blades together.
Return the dumbbells to the starting position while still maintaining the slight bend in your arms.
Repeat for desired number of repetitions (8-12).

Assistance Exercises – Arms

Biceps

Barbell Curls

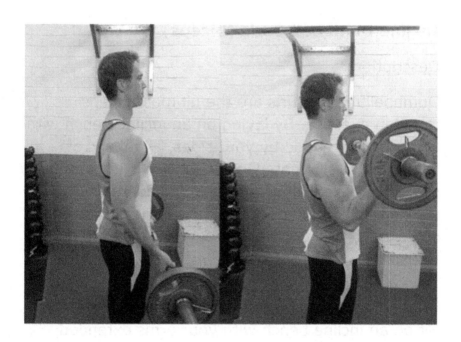

Description:

Barbell curls, the go-to exercise for big arms. Barbell biceps curls are an excellent exercise for adding overall mass to the biceps.

Form:

Stand while holding a barbell with a shoulder width grip – ensure your palms are facing forward.

Keeping your shoulders locked in place, begin to curl the barbell up towards your body by contracting the biceps.
Once biceps are fully contracted, hold and squeeze this position for 1 second.
Slowly lower the bar back to its starting position.
Repeat for the desired number of repetitions (8-12).

Incline Dumbbell Curls (biceps)

Description:

Dumbbell incline curls are the ultimate biceps isolation exercise. By laying on an incline bench with arms fully extended by your sides, all means of cheating are eliminated. Therefore, it is impossible to swing the weight up using your shoulders or momentum. If you perform these curls slowly with strict form, your biceps will feel as if they are ready to explode.

Form:

Sit on an incline bench with your arms extended, holding a dumbbell in each hand.
Lock your shoulders in place, ensuring they don't move for the duration of the exercise.
Curl the dumbbells one at a time up towards your body by contracting the biceps to the fullest extent.
Hold and squeeze the contracted position for 1 second.
Slowly lower each dumbbell back down to your side,

returning your arms to a fully extended position. Repeat for the desired number of repetitions.

Triceps

Barbell Skull Crushers

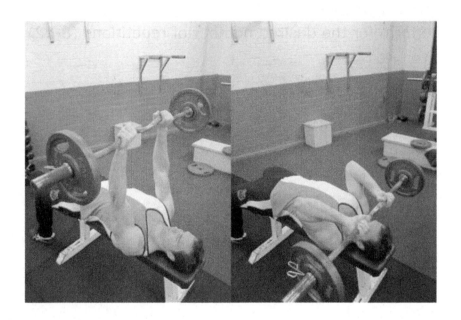

Description:

The barbell skull crusher is a great mass builder for overall size on the 3 heads of the triceps. By ensuring your elbows are as close in as possible and focusing on squeezing the triceps at the top of each repetition, you will experience a pump like no other.

Form:

Lay on a flat bench with a barbell lifted above you. Ensure your arms are straight and your elbows are locked in.

Slowly lower the barbell towards your forehead by moving only your forearms, keeping your elbows locked in place.

Contract the triceps to return the bar back to its starting position.

Perform for the desired number of repetitions (8-12).

Triceps Dips

Description:

Dips form the basis of all triceps routines. Lifting your bodyweight while isolating the triceps is a great overall mass builder. Triceps dips can also be a great means of measuring the triceps strength and progress. Once you've mastered bodyweight triceps dips for 12 repetitions, it's time to start adding additional resistance.

Form:

Hold onto the bars with arms full extended locked above the bars.
While maintaining your body in an upright position and ensuring your elbows stay locked into your sides, begin to lower your body slowly by contracting the triceps.
Continue to lower yourself until a 90 degree angle is formed between your upper arm and forearm.
Push through your triceps to extend your arms back to the starting position.
Repeat for the desired number of repetitions (8-12).

Assistance Exercises – Legs

Leg Press

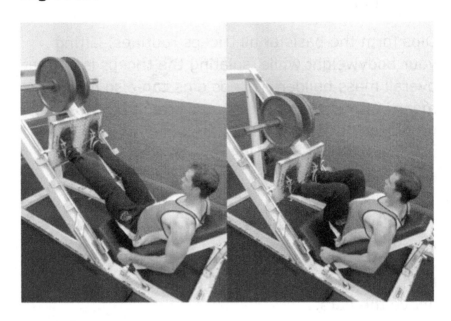

Description:

The leg press is used to add mass and shape to your quads, hamstrings, glutes and calves.
Foot placement on the leg press sled can be manipulated to further target either the quads or hamstrings (higher foot placement targets the hamstrings, while lower foot placement places greater emphasis on the quads).

Form:

Sitting on your leg press machine, place your legs in a shoulder width stance with toes pointing forward

on the leg press sled.
By pressing through your heels, push the platform until your legs are in a locked out position.
Slowly lower the sled until your upper and lower legs form a 90 degree angle.
Once again, push through your heels to return the sled to its starting position.
Repeat for the desired number of repetitions.

Leg Extensions

Description:

Leg extensions are a fantastic quad isolation exercise. The movement is used to develop the 'tear drop' muscle on the quads. To get the most out of leg extensions, focus on the squeeze at the top of each repetition.

Form:

Adjust the leg extension machine to suit your height. Using your quads, extend your legs until they are locked out. Squeeze at the top of each repetition for one second.
Slowly lower the weight back to the original position, without re-racking the weight (ensure you keep tension on your quads for the duration of your set).
Perform for the desired number of repetitions (8-12).

Straight Leg Deadlift

Description:

Straight leg deadlifts (often referred to as stiff leg deadlifts) emphasise the hamstrings and glutes. When performing straight leg deadlifts, you are looking for the deep stretch in the hamstring on each repetition.

Form:

Hold a barbell by your side with your arms fully extended.
Maintain a shoulder width stance.
Keeping your knees locked in place, begin to lower the barbell over the top of your feet. This is achieved by bending at the waist while looking forward to maintain a straight back.
Continue to lower the barbell until you feel a deep stretch in your hamstrings.
Extend your hips and waist to return to the starting position.
Repeat for the desired number of repetitions.

Routines

'Shredded Spartan' Routine – 4 Days per Week

MONDAY - Chest/Back/Biceps

Flat Barbell Bench Press – 5 sets – 3 – 5 repetitions per set. Increase weight each set.

Deadlift – 5 sets – 3 – 5 repetitions per set. Increase weight each set.

Incline Dumbbell Press – 3 sets – 8 – 12 repetitions.

Pull-ups – 3 sets – 8 – 12 repetitions per set (or until failure if you cannot reach 8).

Barbell Curls – 3 sets – 8 -12 repetitions per set.

TUESDAY - Legs/Shoulders/Triceps

Barbell Squats – 5 sets – 3 – 5 repetitions per set. Increase weight each set.

Overhead Press – 5 sets – 3 – 5 repetitions per set. Increase weight each set.

Leg Extensions - 3 sets – 8 – 12 repetitions.

Arnold Dumbbell Press 3 sets – 8 – 12 repetitions.

Triceps Dips 3 sets – 8 – 12 repetitions.

THURSDAY - Chest/Back/Biceps

Flat Barbell Bench Press – 5 sets – 3 – 5 repetitions per set. Increase weight each set.

Deadlift – 5 sets – 3 – 5 repetitions per set. Increase weight each set.

Incline Dumbbell Flyes – 3 sets – 8 – 12 repetitions.

Bent Over Row – 3 sets – 8 – 12 repetitions per set (or until failure if you cannot reach 8).

Incline Dumbbell Curls – 3 sets – 8 -12 repetitions per set.

FRIDAY - Legs/Shoulders/Triceps

Barbell Squats – 5 sets – 3 – 5 repetitions per set. Increase weight each set.

Overhead Press – 5 sets – 3 – 5 repetitions per set. Increase weight each set.

Straight Leg Deadlift - 3 sets – 8 – 12 repetitions.

Dumbbell Lateral Raises - 3 sets – 8 – 12 repetitions.

Triceps Dips - 3 sets – 8 – 12 repetitions.

Advanced
'Shredded Spartan' Routine – 6 Days per Week

MONDAY - Chest/Back

Main Lifts:

Flat Barbell Bench Press – 5 sets – 3 – 5 repetitions per set. Increase weight each set.

Deadlift – 5 sets – 3 – 5 repetitions per set. Increase weight each set.

Assistance Work:

Choose 1 assistance exercise from each of the chest, back and arms (triceps) categories – perform this exercise for 4 sets comprising of 8 – 12 repetitions.

TUESDAY - Legs/Shoulders

Main Lifts:

Barbell Squats – 5 sets – 3 – 5 repetitions per set. Increase weight each set.

Overhead Press – 5 sets – 3 – 5 repetitions per set. Increase weight each set.

Assistance Work:

Choose 1 assistance exercise from each of the chest, back and arms (biceps) categories – perform this exercise for 4 sets comprising of 8 – 12 repetitions.

WEDNESDAY - Chest/Back

Main Lifts:

Flat Barbell Bench Press – 5 sets – 3 – 5 repetitions per set. Increase weight each set.

Deadlift – 5 sets – 3 – 5 repetitions per set. Increase weight each set.

Assistance Work:

Choose 1 assistance exercise from each of the chest, back and arms (triceps) categories – perform this exercise for 4 sets comprising of 8 – 12 repetitions.

THURSDAY - Legs/Shoulders

Main Lifts:

Barbell Squats – 5 sets – 3 – 5 repetitions per set. Increase weight each set.

Overhead Press – 5 sets – 3 – 5 repetitions per set. Increase weight each set.

Assistance Work:

Choose 1 assistance exercise from each of the chest, back and arms (biceps) categories – perform this exercise for 4 sets comprising of 8 – 12 repetitions.

FRIDAY - Chest/Back

Main Lifts:

Flat Barbell Bench Press – 5 sets – 3 – 5 repetitions per set. Increase weight each set.

Deadlift – 5 sets – 3 – 5 repetitions per set. Increase weight each set.

Assistance Work:

Choose 1 assistance exercise from each of the chest, back and arms (triceps) categories – perform this exercise for 4 sets comprising of 8 – 12 repetitions.

SATURDAY - Legs/Shoulders

Main Lifts:

Barbell Squats – 5 sets – 3 – 5 repetitions per set. Increase weight each set.

Overhead Press – 5 sets – 3 – 5 repetitions per set. Increase weight each set.

Assistance Work:

Choose 1 assistance exercise from each of the chest, back and arms (biceps) categories – perform this exercise for 4 sets comprising of 8 – 12 repetitions.

Time Miser
'Shredded Spartan' Routine – 3 Days per Week

Please note: I do not recommend permanently following this routine. The Time Miser Shredded Spartan workout is designed for those periods of time when you just cannot get to the gym the regular 4 – 6 times per week. For example: if you're overseas on a business trip or if you're studying for your final exams – that is the only time I'd recommend you follow this routine... it's not ideal, but it is better than not training.

<u>MONDAY – Full Body</u>

Deadlift - 3 sets – 5 repetitions per set. Increase weight each set.

Bench Press - 3 sets – 5 repetitions per set. Increase weight each set.

Squat - 3 sets – 5 repetitions per set. Increase weight each set.

Overhead Press - 3 sets – 5 repetitions per set. Increase weight each set.

Barbell Curls - 3 sets – 8 – 12 repetitions.

WEDNESDAY – Full Body

Deadlift - 3 sets – 5 repetitions per set. Increase weight each set.

Bench Press - 3 sets – 5 repetitions per set. Increase weight each set.

Squat - 3 sets – 5 repetitions per set. Increase weight each set.

Overhead Press - 3 sets – 5 repetitions per set. Increase weight each set.

Pull-ups - 3 sets – 8 – 12 repetitions.

FRIDAY – Full Body

Deadlift - 3 sets – 5 repetitions per set. Increase weight each set.

Bench Press - 3 sets – 5 repetitions per set. Increase weight each set.

Squat - 3 sets – 5 repetitions per set. Increase weight each set.

Overhead Press - 3 sets – 5 repetitions per set. Increase weight each set.

Tricep Dips - 3 sets – 8 – 12 repetitions.

Spartan Shredded Six Pack Routine

In order to grow our abs, we need to know our abs!

I personally think instead of just doing lots of situps like many beginners do, it is important to know a little bit about the anatomy behind the abs so you can train them effectively.

The abdominals aren't just one muscle – they are made up of a complex group of several muscles.

Rectus Abdominis

The rectus abdominis is a relatively large, flat muscle group located on the front portion of the abdominal wall. It's the most visible abdominal muscle. The rectus abdominis' point of origin is on the pubic crest (hip) bone with cartilage insertion on the fifth through seventh ribs. In terms of movement, the primary functions of the rectus abdominis are to flex the spine forward, to the sides, and to counterbalance spinal extension.

Three lines of tendons, known as tendinous inscriptions, and a white line of connective tissue called the linea alba (literally meaning "white line") separate the rectus into distinct sections, creating its six-pack or washboard appearance.

Obliques

The obliques run alongside that six-pack and taper diagonally into your pants.

The obliques are the masters of trunk rotation (rotate by turning your upper body to the left), but they also factor into spinal flexion, lateral bending, and compressing the abdomen. Twisting exercises are a solid way to target this muscle group and build those sexy side-lines.

Transversus Abdominis

Now we're getting deep into the abdominals. The transversus abdominis isn't a muscle that is visibly defined, so plenty of people don't know it even exists. However, it's been getting more positive attention in recent years, which is a good thing. Not only can including it in your training provide great benefits in overall health and strength, it may also be the abdominal muscle you'd notice most quickly if it was missing. After all, it helps you breathe!

More specifically, contracting the transversus abdominus reduces the diameter of the abdomen. You use it most when you're "belly breathing," sucking in your gut, or forcefully expelling air while making a strong movement like a punch or kick.

When you laugh so hard that you're sore the following day, this is what's tender.

The Exercises

Russian Twists

Russian twists work the upper abdominals and obliques, aim for 20 repetitions per set (10 each side).

Three Quarter Crunch

The three quarter crunch is a classic ab exercise, working the upper middle and lower sections of your abdominals. As we are only doing three quarters of the exercise, this allows us to maintain constant tension on the abs. Perform 15 repetitions in each set.

Planks

Planks work the rectus abdominis as well as the transversus abdominis. These are great for achieving that flat stomach. Hold each plank for at least 30 seconds.

Lying Leg Raises

Leg raises work the entire abdominal region. You can do these lying flat on the floor, or alternatively on a bench (as pictured below).

Perform 15 repetitions per set.

Once these become easy, I would advise performing the advanced version of this exercise – hanging leg raises. The technique is exactly the same, however, it is performed hanging from a pull-up bar.

Ankle Biters

My favourite abdominal exercise! Ankle biters focus on the obliques as they involve a slight twisting movement. I recommend working in a slightly higher repetition range than normal with ankle biters in order to achieve the maximum burn.

Perform 30 repetitions per set, or go to failure if you are unable to reach 30 (which is 15 each side).

Ab Roll Outs

Bonus Exercise – Ab roll outs are fantastic for stressing the entire core. All that is required is an ab roller, and you can pick up one of these on eBay for $10~ including postage, which is a bargain for such a great exercise tool.

Putting it All Together

The heavy main lifts we are performing, including the squat, bench, deadlift and overhead press, all immensely work your core. When you're standing in front of the rack with 400lbs on the bar, your core is what ensures you hold a solid position.

With that said, if you want phenomenal abs that command attention from all who eyes lay upon them, you will still need to perform isolated abdominal work, and that's where the following circuit comes into play.

Perform either 3 sets of each exercise before proceeding onto the next exercise or perform a circuit style workout featuring 1 set of each exercise – if you choose the circuit style method, perform 3 rounds.

I recommend performing this routine 1 – 2 times per week maximum. You can perform it after your workout, or on your rest days. Do not perform this routine before doing your main exercises.

Shredded Spartan Abdominal Annihilation

Russian Twists – 20 reps per set (10 each side)

Three Quarter Sit Ups – 15 reps per set

Planks – 30 second plank

Lying Leg Raises – 15 reps per set

Ankle Biters – 30 reps per set (15 each side)

Ab Roll Outs – 10 reps per set

Diet

You can't out-train a bad diet. Period.

Your diet is king. Without the correct nutrition, your body won't be able to fuel itself in order to become stronger, shred fat and pack on the lean mass you're aiming for after killing it in the gym.

You are to eat like a Spartan. Back in the Spartan and Palaeolithic era, people were lean, energetic and had strong, efficient bodies. Today, with the introduction of fast foods, preservatives and trans fat, the majority of the population, as you know, is overweight, depressed and unhappy – overall, the human race has progressed so far, yet in terms of our diet we've gone backwards.

Your diet will consist solely of the following foods:

Protein Sources:

Chicken

Turkey

Steak

White Fish

Carbohydrate Sources:

Brown Rice

Whole Grain Bread

Sweet Potato

Green Vegetables

Fruits

Fat Sources:

Almonds

Olive Oil (cooking)

Greek Yogurt

Fatty Cuts of Meat

Eggs

Spartans did not graze on food every 2 -3 hours like the majority of fitness magazines and personal trainers recommend you to today. This is a myth that has been debunked - eating small regular meals does NOT increase your metabolism, it does not help you burn any additional fat, so there is absolutely no benefit to doing it.

There's actually a downside...

The human body requires a large amount of energy to effectively digest and process foods. Have you noticed how after a large lunch you're normally quite tired and lethargic (often referred to as a 'food coma')? This is simply due to our body using the majority of our available energy to digest the large meal you've just consumed. By eating small, regular meals, your body will be constantly attempting to break down and digest food, and this is far from efficient.

Spartans do things efficiently...

Spartans hunted for their food; they didn't know whether that meal would be in 2 hours, 2 days or 2 weeks, but when they did acquire food, they had an almighty feast. That is what I recommend you do also, friend.

Eat 2 large meals per day consisting of approved protein, carbohydrate and fat sources.

An example of a Spartan meal plan is as follows:

GET SPARTAN SHREDDED

6:00AM

Wake up

7:00AM

Whey protein shake

12:00PM
Meal 1:

400g scotch fillet steak

2 cups mixed green vegetables

3 eggs

2:00PM

Shredded Spartan Training Regime

5:00PM

15 minute abdominal circuit training

6:00PM
Meal 2:

300g chicken breast

1 cup brown rice

1 handful of roasted almonds

Keep in mind that the above is only a sample. You can adjust your training and meal times to fit around your work or school schedule, however, I advise having a period of no less than 6 hours of fasting between meals 1 and 2.

The macronutrient breakdown of this diet will be roughly 40:30:30. This means that 40% of your daily calories will be consumed via protein, 30% will be consumed via complex carbohydrates, meanwhile the remaining 30% of your daily caloric intake will be consumed via fat.

For an individual aiming to consume 2500 calories per day, their macronutrient breakdown will be as follows:

2500 calories

<u>250 grams of protein</u> (protein contains 4 calories per gram)

<u>188 grams of carbohydrates</u> (carbohydrates contain 4 calories per gram)

<u>83 grams of fat</u> (fat contains 9 calories per gram)

Breakdown calculated using macronutrientcalculator.com

'So how do I know how many calories my body needs each day?'

Here's the magical formula:

For men

BMR = [9.99 x weight (kg)] + [6.25 x height (cm)] - [4.92 x age (years)] + 5

The above equation will give you your BMR – this is your Basal Metabolic Rate. In other words, the number of calories your body needs to function while at rest.

You then multiply the BMR by an 'activity variable' to obtain your TDEE (total daily energy expenditure). This Activity Factor is the cost of living and it is based on more than just your workouts. It also includes work/lifestyle, sports, and the thermogenic effect of food (essentially the amount of energy burned in the process of digesting food).

Average activity variables are as follows:

1.2 = Sedentary - Little or no exercise + desk job

1.3-1.4 = Lightly Active - Little daily activity and light exercise 1-3 days a week

1.5-1.6 = Moderately Active - Moderately active daily life and moderate exercise 3-5 days a week

1.7-1.8 = Very Active - Physically demanding lifestyle and hard exercise or sports 6-7 days a week

1.9-2.0 = Extremely Active - Hard daily exercise or sports and physical job

Below are some examples of this calculation performed correctly:

90kg male – 21 years old - 187cm tall – desk job, minimal exercise

[9.99 * 90] + [6.25 * 187] – [4.92 * 21] – 5 * Activity Level 1.2 = 2350 calories

70kg male – 18 years old - 170cm tall – physical job, lots of exercise

[9.99 * 70] + [6.25 * 170] – [4.92 * 18] – 5 * Activity level 1.7 = 2852 calories

Once you have acquired your magical caloric intake number, all you need to do is either add an additional 500 calories if you wish to bulk (add more mass, while gaining minimal fat) or cut (get shredded, sculpted abs and reveal your chest and arm vascularity by burning off unnecessary fat you're currently holding).

Just to ensure you grasp the concept:

BMR * Activity Level = caloric intake

Caloric intake + 500 = bulking caloric intake

Caloric intake − 500 = cutting caloric intake

Supplementation

Fitness supplements are a multi-billion dollar industry – but do all the supplements on the market do what they claim? Certainly not. No powder will 'Increase your bench press by 128% as proven by college studies' or give you the 'ripped abs you deserve, in 3 weeks or less.' If it sounds too good to be true, it probably is. Supplements serve the purpose they suggest: they simply 'supplement' your diet. Provided you are hitting your caloric intake and macronutrients each day, supplementation may contribute up to 5%.

Back in the day, Spartans did not have access to all the fancy supplements available today, but, like I mentioned, you can use them to get that slight edge.

As long as newcomers continue to get conned into purchasing all of these magical powders and pills, the supplementation industry will continue to thrive. Did you know that many supplements don't even undergo any testing or approval before they are allowed to be sold on the shelves?

The supplements listed below are ones I have been personally using for years and would recommend incorporating into your Shredded Spartan routine. These are the basics, and they have been proven true, unlike many of the other supplements full of fluff and filler ingredients that are on the market.

GET SPARTAN SHREDDED

Protein

The primary purpose of protein powder is to assist you in reaching your macronutrient breakdown, and, depending on your daily intake, it can be hard (and time consuming) to get your protein intake for the day in via solid food – this is where protein powder comes in to play. 1 scoop of protein powder has between 25 and 30 grams of protein.

Protein is protein. It doesn't vary as much between brands as the manufacturers will lead you to believe. No protein is twice as effective as another, so why should you pay twice as much? Keep it simple and get the right type of protein as opposed to focusing on the brand.

WPI (Whey Protein Isolate)
Whey Protein Isolate is a fast acting type of protein. It begins working almost immediately and is best suited to a post-workout meal. It has no other place in your diet.

WPC (Whey Protein Concentrate)
This is a much cheaper version of WPI, and acts over a much longer period of time. This can be used at any time, but still doesn't compare to, for example, egg protein, as far as effectiveness. WPC is a lot cheaper than WPI and is almost as good; it really provides value for the money.

Casein Protein (Slow Release)

This is a slow acting protein, and generally lasts about 5 hours in your system. This is ideal before bed, or for a midnight snack. If you have the budget, I'd purchase some of this just to take before bed as it will fuel your body for quite some time.

Multivitamin

Multivitamins can greatly help your diet. They're ideal for helping to supplement the vitamins and minerals that your body is deficient in. Some of these you could possibly miss by having a flexible diet. When putting together a diet, we quite often limit how much variety we have. This will lead to us neglecting vital vitamins. The best way to take care of this is simply taking a decent multivitamin. Most of them on the market are fairly priced and provide you with everything you will need from vitamin B to Zinc.

Fish Oil

Fish oil contains EFA (essential fatty acids). It is available in both capsule and liquid form and has many benefits, including a healthier blood cholesterol profile and improved bone health – no more squeaky joints! It also assists in protecting against major diseases, such as cancer. Fish oil also assists in increasing the serotonin levels within your body which results in an overall increase in happiness and well-being. Recent studies also show that fish oil may have an influence on muscle protein synthesis.

When selecting fish oil, ensure they are high in EPA/DHA as these are the main omega 3 fatty acids.

I recommend consuming between 2 – 3G per day (capsules generally come in 1000mg and 1500mg).

Vitamin C

No other vitamin has as many positive effects on the body as vitamin C. As vitamin C is not stored in your body, it needs to be replenished daily. Without supplementation, reaching your daily vitamin C intake can be quite difficult.

Vitamin C is required for the growth and repair of tissues in all parts of your body. It is used to form collagen, a protein used to make skin, scar tissue, tendons, ligaments, and blood vessels. It is also essential for the healing of wounds, and for the repair and maintenance of your cartilage, bones, and teeth. Vitamin C also helps with blood pressure by strengthening the walls of your arteries. It can also prevent damage to cells caused by aging as well as help reduce levels of stress.

For athletes, vitamin C will keep testosterone levels high by supporting a lower ratio of cortisol to testosterone. This will help your body keep up that top level of performance you require on a daily basis.

I recommend consuming 1g of vitamin C per day. As vitamin C is water soluble, any excess amount of this vitamin will simply be urinated out within 24 hours.

Caffeine/Coffee

Caffeine is an alkaloid compound found in the seeds, leaves and fruits of various plants. Caffeine is a mild stimulant and drug that acts upon the brain and central nervous system. According to The New York Times, caffeine is known as "the most popular drug used in sports today." Caffeine is apparent in coffee, tea, and pre-workout supplements and capsules to name a few variations.

Caffeine has been involved with many studies over the years, reinforcing its positive effects in fat loss, mental focus and overall physical performance.

The greatest benefit of having caffeine before your workout is its fat burning properties. High amounts of caffeine in black coffee will increase your metabolism, which makes you burn more calories throughout the day. Having coffee before exercise enhances that effect. Also, caffeine and other compounds found in coffee act as an appetite suppressant, making you consume less overall.

Several studies have demonstrated a link between caffeine intake before exercise and increased athletic performance. A report published in *Sports Medicine* refers to caffeine as a "powerful ergogenic aid," and mentions that athletes can "train at a greater power output and/or train longer" after caffeine consumption. Another study published in the *British Journal of Sports Science* found that subjects who consumed coffee before running 1500 meters on the treadmill completed their run 4.2 seconds faster than the control group, on average. To gain an extra edge in your training sessions, coffee might be just what you need.

Along with increased energy to push through tough workouts, caffeine provides an increase in mental focus as well. Improved focus will help keep workouts productive and effective.

Researchers at the University of Illinois found that subjects who consumed caffeine prior to exercise experienced less muscle pain during their workout than their non-caffeinated counterparts. What conclusion can we draw from this? You can complete more reps at a higher resistance during your weight training sessions, and run faster and longer during your cardio workouts with the assistance of caffeine.

Consuming caffeine in the form of coffee helps protect your body from diseases. Coffee contains large amounts of antioxidants, which protect against damage from free radicals. According to a 2011 study published in *Critical Reviews in Food Science and Nutrition*, coffee consumption has an inverse correlation with diabetes, Parkinson's disease, Alzheimer's disease, and certain forms of cancer.

I recommend consuming 200 – 300mg of caffeine before your workouts (in the form of black coffee), however, individuals have different stimulant tolerances. I would experiment with various doses, but do not exceed this amount. It is beneficial to 'cycle' caffeine as the human body quickly builds a tolerance to the stimulant properties of caffeine and will, therefore, not be as effective. A 1:1 on:off ratio works well.

Training Aids

In order to achieve a Shredded Spartan physique and super-human strength, you do not require any specific equipment besides a gym membership and the desire to achieve what you've set your mind to.

However, there are a few useful pieces of equipment that I do personally use and recommend – keep in mind that with these products there is no specific brand I recommend; all these products are basic, so if you choose to purchase any of them, don't fall for the marketing hype and pay twice as much as you should for a basic leather belt or material straps. Be a Spartan, think smart.

Wrist Straps

Wrist straps come in handy for heavy pulling exercises such as the deadlift, bent over row, pull-ups and even barbell curls. The primary function of wrist straps is to allow you to train the targeted muscle group (e.g. back) even after your grip strength has degraded, as the majority of the time when performing a pulling exercise, such as the deadlift, your grip will reach failure before your back – straps assist your grip and therefore lets you squeeze out those last few reps.

There are 2 variations of straps available: 'regular' straps which you loop around the bar and then grip onto, the other version being 'figure 8' straps, figure

8 straps are comprised of two loops – one loop is to be wrapped around your wrist while the other is wrapped around the barbell, pulling to tighten the grip.

I personally use figure 8 straps due to ease of use – this is, however, is simply my personal preference. Both are cheap, effective and will provide the same result.

Weightlifting Belt

Weightlifting belts are designed to take the pressure off your lower back and abdominal region while you are performing your main compound lifts, primarily the squat and deadlift. Many people train consistently with a belt, but I do not recommend this. A weight belt should only be used on extremely heavy sets, such as when you're trying to break a personal record or when you are performing your last set or two of your main lift. Constant reliance on a weightlifting belt will result in a weak core which can increase your risk of injury later down the track.

Gym Chalk

Weightlifting chalk can be used as a substitute for straps. Weightlifting chalk, when applied thoroughly to your hands, will accelerate your grip and forearm development, allowing you to grip onto the barbell comfortably during your last few repetitions of heavy deadlifts. However, here is a word of warning: many gyms do not appreciate members using chalk as it can be quite messy if you're not careful when you're applying and storing it. I personally do not use chalk often; however, it definitely is worth mentioning as a training aid. I recommend checking if chalk is allowed at your local gym (chances are if you train at a large chain gym, such as Planet Fitness, it will be).

Weighted Belts

Weighted belts are great for those advanced Spartan trainers. A weighted belt is essentially a leather belt with a looped chain and carabineer that allows you to fasten additional weight to your belt in order to increase the load and difficulty of bodyweight exercises, such as the pull-up and tricep dip. If you can perform 12+ repetitions of the pull-up or tricep dip during your accessory exercises for 3 or more consecutive sets, it's time to consider investing in a weighted belt or vest. Alternatively, you can hold a dumbbell between your legs. (I personally find it quite hard to hold a dumbbell between my legs once going past 20lb of additional weight as it tends to fall out of place after a few repetitions, but it may work for you! Give it a try before investing in a weighted belt.)

Motivation

Let's take a look at motivation. Motivation is something inside of you; you can teach and express the importance of motivation, but unless an individual is motivated, they will not follow through with anything. You must remain motivated to train; you have to want it bad... and for the right reasons too.

There are two types of motivation:

Internal Motivation

Internal motivation is pure and self-created. Internal motivation to perform any given task is apparent because this task is in line with your personal values and goals.

An example of internal motivation:

I want to get in the best shape of my life in order to lower my risk and disease, increase my confidence and prove to myself that I can achieve whatever I set my mind to.

External Motivation

External motivation is when the only reason you are aiming to achieve the given task is due to a reward, which is more often than not monetary. External motivation is not sustainable as you will be unable to give your full effort to tasks which you are not being compensated for.

An example of external motivation:

A classic example of external motivation is attempting to get in the best shape of your life so you can win the prize money at your local bodybuilding competition. If you're doing it for the money, you'll never be able to make it through the tough times.

In order to stay motivated, set clear cut goals. Do you want to lift a certain amount of weight by the end of this year? Do you want to look a certain way? Have a single digit level of body fat perhaps?

Align your actions with your goals

The next step is ensuring everything you do aligns with these goals.

Next time you go to buy fast food or skip the gym, ask yourself, "Is what I'm about to do bringing me closer or further away from the person I want to become?" If the answer is yes, proceed. If the answer is no, then you know you shouldn't be doing it. It's all a matter of will, and it really is that simple.

Before you hit the gym

Before your training session, in order to get yourself amped up and motivated to demolish the weights like a true Spartan, I recommend creating yourself a gym playlist on your iPod that gets you fired up and in the mood to lift – this comes down to personal preference. Some peoples playlist may consist of heavy metal or rap while others will prefer electronic style music. Whatever you choose, ensure it gets you fired up to lift.

If you're feeling tired or just want to truly get in the zone for your training session, I recommend consuming a strong black coffee between 15 – 30 minutes prior to your workout. As mentioned above in the supplementation section, caffeine found in black coffee has many benefits – one of these being its ability to assist with an increase in mental focus to push you through those tough workouts. You will be efficient and productive like a true Spartan.

"Champions come in pairs of 2 because they battle each other into perfection." – Greg Plitt

True Spartans never fight alone, the same goes in the gym – if you want the ultimate motivation, find yourself a dedicated training partner that is committed to training with you day in and day out. You will push each other to levels you would not be able to reach alone by encouraging each other to push out those last few reps. You will also be able to assist your training partner by spotting them on crucial lifts, such as the bench press, to really get the maximum bang for your buck and help you lift weight you didn't think would be possible on your own.

Tracking Progression

"In order to know where we're going we must first know where we are and where we have been." – Greg Plitt

When you get in your car, you have an end destination in mind, along with check points on the way to this destination. In your weight loss/mass gain diet, these progress checks are your check points, while your dream body is the destination.

Tracking progress is essential. Without regularly checking your progress, you won't know whether your current training regime and caloric intake are suitable for you.

Most individuals simply rely on the scales to track progress; don't fall into the trap of weighing yourself daily. Remember: weight constantly fluctuates based on the time of the day as well as other factors, such as fluid intake, meals consumed, stress and a number of other factors. Therefore, I personally deem the methods below, along with a weigh in on the scales once a week (first thing in the morning prior to consuming any food), to be the most accurate way to determine whether you're making progress.

Realistic expectations - I am not here to tell you that you're going to lose 20kg of fat in 5 weeks, or that you can stack on lean muscle in a few days of hitting your caloric goal. These results are simply not attainable. Consistent results are the best kind of results. Following a ketogenic or low carbohydrate diet will initially give you a large period of weight loss as this is the process of your body losing water weight due to a decrease in carbohydrates (as water binds to carbohydrates). But, soon after that, the progress will diminish. Please refer to the following figures which are ideal for consistent fat loss.

Body Composition	Estimated Consistent Loss
Lean (<15%)	1lb per week
Average (15 – 20%)	2lbs per week
Overweight (>20%)	4lbs per week

Measurements

Use a tape measure and measure the circumference of your neck, chest, biceps, waist, thighs and calves. Record these measurements in a Microsoft Excel spread sheet weekly. Here is an example:

Body Part	Week 1	Week 2	Week 3
Neck (circumference, cm)	42cm	41cm	40.5cm
Chest	68cm	68cm	69cm
Biceps (average of 2)	35cm	35cm	36cm
Waist	80cm	79cm	77cm
Thighs (average of 2)	60cm	59cm	58.5cm
Calves (average of 2)	40cm	40cm	40cm

Based on the example table above, you can see that the sizes of this individuals arms and chest are increasing, while their waist and thighs have slowly started to decrease. Tracking progress via these measurements allows us to see which body parts are progressing and which are lagging behind – adjustments to your routine can then be made to counteract this.

Photos

Take photos of your physique on a weekly basis, including front, side and rear views of your physique. When taking these progress photos, ensure they are taken in the same location at the same time of day consistently (I would recommend first thing in the morning) to avoid any differences in lighting and water retention from food, etc. This is to ensure you capture the most accurate representation of your physique each time – making it easy to gauge progress. Print out these photos and stick them on your bathroom mirror; record your weight and body measurements on the back. There is no better motivation then seeing your hard work transform into progress.

Body Fat Percentage

If you have access to a body fat caliper, it is recommended you also measure your body fat percentage every 2 weeks. Body fat calipers can be purchased online for as little as $4 and come with full instructions on how to accurately measure your body fat. The most common and accurate sites to measure from include your pectoral, triceps, lats, lower abdomen and thigh.

Others methods used to measure your body fat percentage include:

Body fat scales - An electric current is pulsed through your body and uses biometrical impedance analysis to analyze the amount of body fat you are holding. I would not recommend using this method as the result given can vary dramatically based on the amount of water you are holding.

The measurement method - By taking measurements using the US Navy body fat calculating technique, you can calculate your body fat percentage. A link to calculate your body fat using this method is located in the 'Useful Links' section at the end of this book.

DEXA Scanning- DEXA scanning is undoubtedly the most accurate method as it takes a full X-ray of your body composition and gives you the numbers. DEXA scans are performed at specialized health clinics; the process of getting a DEXA scan involves you lying on an X-Ray table for 15 minutes. It's typically very expensive, coming in at around the $200 mark, although, as stated, it is the most accurate method.

Looking

If you are familiar with what a male or female body looks like at certain body fat levels, you can simply gauge where you are currently in comparison. A chart below showing both male and female physiques at different body fat percentages will assist you if this is the method you choose to use.

This, however, is not the method I recommend for measuring ongoing progress (as if you lose 1% body fat over the course of a week or two, it can be hard to distinguish from simply looking). That is where a caliper is best used.

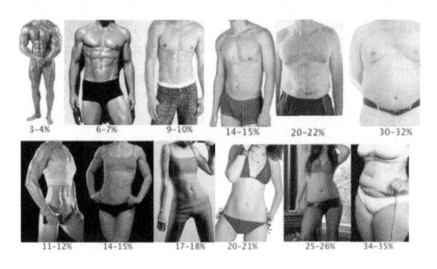

Clothing

That favourite shirt of yours that you want to fill out or those jeans you haven't been able to comfortably fit in for the last couple of years are a great way to gauge your progress. Over time, you will start to see the composition of your body change. If you're adding lean mass, you will notice your shirts start to fit tighter around the arms. Your shoulder will fill out the shirt more as your waist begins to decrease in circumference.

Recording your lifts

I also recommend investing in a simple notepad to document your workouts. Record the number of reps and sets you performed at each weight during your workout, then as you begin to struggle happen to lose motivation, you can look back upon your journey and reflect on what was working, what wasn't working, what you have done and perhaps where you should go from here. Don't go through your workouts blindly – record them.

Conclusion

Thank you again for purchasing this book!

Now you know how to train, eat, recover, supplement and stay motivated like a true Spartan Warrior. By following the diet and training regime I have documented for you in this book, you'll not only build the body of your dreams, but you will also unknowingly build unbreakable confidence, pride and determination. Your mind will reflect your body and you will be unstoppable – any dreams, any goals, any aspirations will suddenly all be within reach.

There is no better feeling in this world then progressively getting closer and closer to your dream body each and every day.

Now that you've got the information, it's time to implement it and take massive action! Ditch your old workout regime and diet that gave you mediocre results and get started on your path to become a shredded Spartan Warrior today.

Finally, if you enjoyed this book, please take the time to share your thoughts and post a review on Amazon. It'd be greatly appreciated!

Thank you and best of luck with your journey.

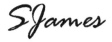

Glossary

1RM

1 rep maximum, the heaviest amount of weight you are able to lift with correct form for 1 repetition.

AAS

Short for anabolic-androgenic steroids. These drugs have similar effects to testosterone within the body. Protein in cells - specifically in skeletal muscles are increased with the aid of AAS.

Abdominals

The muscle group located between the chest and pelvis, responsible for stabilising the body. The abdominal region is made up of the rectus abdominis, external obliques, intercoastals, serratus and TVA.

Basal Metabolic Rate

The number of calories your body expends while at rest.

Biceps

Technically known as the biceps brachii, a two headed muscle located between the elbow and shoulder.

Body Fat

The total amount of fat you are carrying on your body, measured as a percentage.

Body Mass Index

Often referred to as BMI, body mass index is a measure used to roughly calculate the amount of fat you are carrying based on your gender, height and weight. BMI is measured within ranges.

Bulking

The process of consuming a larger amount of calories than your total daily energy expenditure in an effort to gain additional muscle mass.

Caffeine

An alkaloid compound commonly found in tea and coffee plants.
Caffeine is a stimulant of the CNS.

Calorie

A unit of heat used to indicate the amount of energy that a food will produce in the human body.The human body requires a certain caloric intake simply in order to survive.

Carbohydrate

An organic compound comprised of carbon, hydrogen and oxygen.
4 calories per gram.

Cardio

Cardiovascular exercise, also referred to as aerobic exercise. Cardio is used to increase the heart rate in order to burn calories, cardio is typically performed for an extended period of time at 60 – 85% of the individuals maximum heart rate.

Calves

The rear portion of the lower leg.
The calf muscle attaches to the heel via the Achilles tendon.

CNS

Acronym for Central Nervous System.
The nervous system consisting of the spinal cord and brain.

Cutting

Cutting is the process of shedding bodyfat in order to reveal lean muscle mass, cutting is achieved via being in a calorie deficit for a prolonged period of time.

Deltoids

The muscle that forms a rounded contour of the shoulder.
The deltoids are made up of 3 heads, the anterior (front) deltoid the lateral (side) deltoid and the posterior (rear) deltoid.

DOMS

Acronym for delayed onset muscle soreness, the pain and stiffness that generally occurs 24 – 72 hours after exercising the particular muscle.

Drop Set

An advanced lifting technique involving decreasing the weight of an exercise to a lighter weight immediately after reaching failure to promote further growth.

Equipment

Barbells, skipping ropes, squat racks etc. anything that is primarily used for exercise.

External Motivation

Motivation with an incentive for reaching the end goal.

Fat

Natural oil like substance deposited under the skin.

Gear

A slang term for AAS.

Giant Set

3 or more exercises performed back to back without any rest period inbetween – a giant set can be performed on an individual muscle, or can target opposing muscles (e.g. chest and back).

HIIT

High intensity interval training. A short duration form of cardio that alternates between periods of low intensity (recovery) aerobic exercise with bursts of intense aerobic exercise.

Hypertrophy

Hypertrophy is the process of increasing the size of muscle cells.

Hamstrings

Tendons that attach the muscle on the rear of the leg (thigh) to the bone.
The hamstring muscle pulls on these tendons.

Insulin Spike

An insulin spike is the increase of the hormone insulin secreted by the pancreas as a result of an increase in blood sugar. An insulin spike is accomplished by eating foods with a high glycaemic index.

IF

Acronym for intermittent fasting – a style of diet that is based around 1 or 2 large meals per day with an 8+ fast in between eating windows.

Internal Motivation

A form of motivation created within in order to achieve a higher task.

LISS

Low intensity sustained state, a form of aerobic cardio that involves performing a gentle form of cardio e.g. walking for an extended period of time, generally 45 minutes or more.

Locking Out

When lifting, hyper extending the arms or legs so the weight being lifted is transferred onto the joints and tendons at the top of each repetition and is no longer keeping tension on the muscle.

Macronutrients

The breakdown of protein, carbohydrate and fats found in all foods.

Metabolism

A chemical process that occurs within your body required to maintain life.

Micronutrients

Beneficial chemical elements and traces found in foods that are required for growth and life.

Mind Muscle Connection

The signal sent from the brain to the targeted muscle in order for it to contract, this occurs at the neuromuscular junction. A chemical neurotransmitter known as Acetylcholine is released by the brain to communicate with the muscle.

Mineral

A naturally occurring substance that is solid at room temp.

Muscle

Fibrous tissue within the body that has the ability to contract in order to produce movement.

Natural

An individual whom has not used AAS or any other hormone altering compounds to increase muscle mass or decrease body fat.

Posterior Chain

The posterior chain is a group of muscles comprised of the hamstrings, glutes and lower back, a solid posterior chain is required for almost all athletic activities.

PR

Personal record, often also referred to as personal best.
Often used when discussing your 1 rep maximum.

Priority Training

Identifying and targeting muscle groups on your physique that are lagging behind the others. An example of priority training is training chest twice a week for an individual whom is lacking overall chest thickness.

Processed

A food or object that has undergone chemical operations to preserve it.

Protein

A nutrient required by the human body for both growth and performance.

Pump

The feeling of muscular tightness after training a muscle. The pump is the result of blood engorging the muscle.

Quads

Short for quadriceps, the four headed muscle located on the front of the upper leg. The quadriceps are the extensor of the knee.

Refeed

A refeed is the process of re-filling muscle glycogen stores after following a low carbohydrate diet for a period of time. During a refeed period carbohydrate intake is greatly increased.

ROM

Acronym for range of motion, the movement and contraction of the muscle.

Stimulant

Substance responsible for increasing both mental and physical functions for a temporary period of time.

Super Set

An advanced training technique comprised of performing 2 exercises back to back without any rest between. Supersets can be performed for the same or opposing muscle groups.

Supplement

An extra element or substance consumed to gain an upper hand.

Total Daily Energy Expenditure

Often referred to as TDEE, the number of calories your body needs to consume in order to maintain its current state at your current activity level, also known as your maintenance calorie level.

Thermic Effect of Food

Often referred to as TEF, the thermic effect of food is the number of calories expended by consuming and digesting food.

Triceps

The muscle group located on the posterior of the arm between the shoulder and the elbow, the triceps are responsible for straightening of the arm – the triceps are made up of 3 heads known as the long head, the lateral head and the medial head.

Vitamin

A vitamin is an organic nutritional substance often found in small quantities.

Made in the USA
Middletown, DE
26 November 2021

53513314R00066